The Natural Way to a Healthy Prostate

Preventing prostate problems with nutritional and herbal treatments

Michael B. Schachter, M.D.

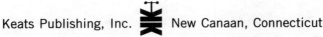

Keats Publishing, Inc. New Canaan, Connecticut

ABOUT THE AUTHOR

Michael B. Schachter, M.D., a graduate of the Columbia College of Physicians and Surgeons, has been practicing complementary medicine since 1974, most recently in Suffern, New York. He is regarded as one of the nation's leading practitioners in alternative cancer therapy. He is also certified in chelation therapy by the American Board of Chelation Therapy. Dr. Schachter has been active in many complementary medicine groups and is a former president of the American College for Advancement in Medicine and current president of the Foundation for the Advancement of Innovative Medicine (FAIM). He is the author (with the late Dr. David Sheinkin and Richard Hutton) of *The Food Connection* and *Food, Mind and Mood*, in addition to many articles on various aspects of complementary medicine.

The author gratefully acknowledges the assistance of Toby Hindin, M.S., C.N.S., for her invaluable help in editing this manscript.

The Natural Way to a Healthy Prostate is not intended as medical advice. Its intent is solely informational and educational. Please consult a health professional should the need for one be indicated.

Good Health Guides are published by
Keats Publishing, Inc.
27 Pine Street (Box 876)
New Canaan, Connecticut 06840-0876

Contents

INTRODUCTION

The prostate gland, an essential part of the male reproductive system, is necessary for reproduction and sexual functioning. Yet, it also sets the stage for a variety of serious health problems. The purpose of this book is to describe the major health problems associated with the prostate; how these problems are generally handled by conventional medicine; and most importantly, how you can prevent these problems from developing or manage them if they are already present using noninvasive, natural and relatively nontoxic methods.

Some of the ideas presented are highly controversial, and the reader is encouraged to seek medical evaluation and opinion for any prostate problem with both a conventional physician, such as a urologist, and a complementary physician. A complementary physician is one who is familiar with both conventional and alternative approaches to medical problems. It is essential that the reader question any physician in detail before undergoing any procedure or treatment. The risks and benefits of the therapy should be crystal clear.

The major health problems associated with the prostate may be divided into three main categories: (1) enlargement of the prostate, often called benign prostatic hyperplasia, or BPH; (2) prostatitis or inflammation of the prostate; and (3) prostate cancer. The human pain and financial cost of these conditions are astronomical. It has been estimated that the prostate gland accounts for more than 5.5 million doctor visits, 950,000 hospitalizations and 43,500 prostate-related deaths per year, all at a national cost of over $7 billion. It is time for the public to become more aware of the problems associated with the prostate gland and how to prevent or treat them.

THE PROSTATE GLAND

The prostate gland is not exactly a gland at all, but an organ that contains about 70 percent glandular tissue and 30 percent fibromuscular tissue. It is a small chestnut-shaped organ situated directly beneath the male bladder and in front of the rectum. It is surrounded by a thick fibrous capsule. In an adult, it weighs about 20 grams.

From birth until puberty, very little growth of the prostate takes place. At puberty, the prostate itself undergoes a growth spurt, increasing in weight and doubling its size. In general, the size of the prostate remains constant for the next several years. In some men, in fact, the prostate never again increases in size. Unfortunately, however, this is not the case for most men, who will develop benign prostatic hypertrophy in their forties, fifties or sixties.

The urethra is a flexible tube that connects the bladder with the outside. From the bladder, the urethra passes directly through the center of the prostate en route to the penis. The portion of the urethra that passes through the prostate is called the prostatic urethra. From the end of the prostate, the urethra passes longitudinally through the shaft of the penis. The urethra has two functions—to transport urine and to transport semen. During urination, the fibromuscular tissue of the prostate actively contracts to dilate the prostatic urethra, allowing urine to flow from the bladder to the penis and then to the outside.

Urine originates in the kidneys, the excretory organs located in the mid- to lower back region. From each kidney, a narrow flexible tube, called a ureter, carries urine to the bladder. These ureters, which transport urine from the kidneys to the bladder, should not be confused with the single urethra, which carries urine from the bladder to the penis and out of the body.

From the bladder, the prostatic urethra ends at the external sphincter, the muscle that you voluntarily contract when you are urinating and want to stop the flow suddenly. At the other end of the prostatic urethra closest to the bladder is another sphincter, called the internal sphincter. It operates involuntarily to prevent semen from discharging into the bladder during ejaculation. Under certain circumstances, when the urethra is partially blocked due to an enlarged prostate, the pressure that builds up in the bladder may cause a reflux of urine back into the ureters. This may result in chronically dilated ureters, which may lead to chronic kidney disease, a condition which ultimately may be fatal.

The second function of the urethra involves the transportation of semen during ejaculation. The prostate glandular tissue secretes a fluid that contributes to the seminal fluid carrying spermatozoa. The combination of spermatozoa, seminal vesicle fluid and prostatic fluid, in addition to a tiny amount of fluid from some minor glands, constitute semen. The prostate gland fluid, a thin, milky substance, is secreted into the urethra during ejaculation. This fluid is what gives semen its characteristic odor. Contents of these secretions include calcium, zinc, citric acid, acid phosphatase, albumin and prostatic specific antigen. These substances aid in the lubrication of the urethra and the protection, nourishment and motility of sperm in the acid environment of the vagina. Initially produced during sexual excitement, prostatic fluid constitutes approximately 20 percent of the volume of semen.

Endocrine Glands and Hormones

Endocrine hormones are substances secreted by glands into the bloodstream. Hormones can influence physiological processes far from the location of the glands that secrete them. Examples of endocrine glands are the pituitary, thyroid, adrenals, the testes in men and the ovaries in women.

The testes produce male sex hormones, a subtype of steroids called androgens, the most important of which are testosterone and dihydrotestosterone or DHT. Some of the testosterone travels through the bloodstream to the prostate gland, where much of it is converted to dihydrotestosterone, as a result of the action of the enzyme 5-alpha reductase. This is an irreversible reaction.

However, not all of the testosterone entering the prostate is converted to dihydrotestosterone. A small amount is converted to the female sex steroid, estradiol by action of the enzyme aromatase. Knowledge of DHT and 5-alpha reductase is important in understanding both normal and pathologic prostate conditions.

BENIGN DISORDERS OF THE PROSTATE

BENIGN PROSTATIC HYPERPLASIA (BPH)

Benign prostatic hyperplasia, formerly called benign prostatic hypertrophy (abbreviated BPH), is a nonmalignant enlargement of the prostate. Both the glandular and the muscular or connective tissue elements of the prostate may increase in size. "Benign" affirms that the condition is nonmalignant or noncancerous. "Hypertrophy" means increased in size, and "hyperplasia" refers to an increase in cells. BPH is very common in men over 40 years of age in all races and cultures. However, men usually do not notice any symptoms until age 50 or beyond.

According to estimates by the American Foundation for Urologic Disease, more than half of men aged 50 and above have enlarged prostates. The number steadily increases with age, and by age 80, about 80 percent of men have prostatic enlargement. Half of these men have symptoms of BPH, and about one-quarter of these symptomatic men will undergo surgery to alleviate symptoms. Approximately 10 percent of all men in the United States will have prostate surgery at some point in their lives. The chance of experiencing BPH increases with age. The two conditions that seem to be necessary, but not necessarily sufficient, for the development of BPH in men are increased age and the presence of DHT.

Benign prostatic hyperplasia is generally described as an increase in the number of cells of the transitional zone of the prostate, the prostatic zone that surrounds the urethra. Enlargement in this zone may cause symptoms of urinary tract blockage. As the prostate tissue enlarges, it may compress the prostatic urethra, impeding the flow of urine through its normal route. This results in symptoms of urinary-flow impairment.

For the past fifty years, when this condition became bad enough, it was treated with surgery involving the removal of extra tissue impinging on the prostatic urethra. This operation is called a TURP, or transurethral resection of the prostate. Approximately 400,000 such resections are performed annually in the United States, making this operation the second most common after cataract extraction in men older than 65. The annual cost in the United States for treatment of this condition is approximately $5 billion. Surgical treatment for BPH is on the wane, as drug therapy is beginning to be used as a possible substitute.

BPH can be identified by symptoms of the patient, findings on physical examination by the physician and certain tests. However, the major clues to the diagnosis are the symptoms.

Symptoms of BPH

The symptoms may be divided into two categories: (1) urinary obstruction symptoms and (2) bladder irritability symptoms. Obstructive symptoms may include a decrease in the force of the urine stream, hesitancy (trouble initiating the urine stream), dribbling (trouble shutting off the urine stream) and a feeling of bladder fullness even after voiding. This feeling of fullness is generally due to actual urinary retention, which occurs because the urine remaining in the bladder toward the end of urination does not have the force necessary to shoot itself through an obstructed urethra.

Irritative symptoms may result from BPH, from the inflammation and infection of prostatitis or from cancer of the prostate gland. These include dysuria (painful urination), frequent urges to urinate and a feeling of urgency that may precede voiding.

BPH often can go undetected initially because the muscle in the bladder wall (the detrusor muscle) may compensate for the resistance to urine flow by increasing in size (hypertrophy). On cystoscopic examination, during which the bladder may be visualized directly by the urologist, the hypertrophic changes in the muscles of the bladder wall are called trabeculation. Symptoms of obstruction will then not be experienced until the blockage becomes so severe that even the compensatory hypertrophy of the detrusor muscle will not be sufficient to aid in emptying the bladder.

As a BPH condition worsens, the amount of urine retained in the bladder increases, and additional symptoms and signs may occur. These include nocturia (waking up during the night to urinate) and incontinence (the inability to prevent urination). Rarely, the prostate will enlarge posteriorly and cause obstruction of the rectum and constipation.

The relationship between the degree of hyperplasia and obstruction of the urethra is not direct. In other words, sometimes men have BPH but remain symptom free. Conversely, there can be severe obstruction of the urethra even when the hyperplasia has not increased the size of the gland past normal limits. In fact, a significant percentage of TURP surgeries performed to alleviate alleged impingement of the prostate on the urinary tract are performed on individuals with a normal-sized prostate.

Prostatism and the American Urologic Association Index

The symptoms associated with prostate dysfunction are often termed prostatism. Although most often associated with BPH, they may also be caused by dysfunction of the urethral sphincters, bladder muscle dysfunction, prostatitis and prostate cancer. In 1992, the American Urologic Association published a questionnaire designed for physicians to give to patients to help to quantify prostatism. Although originally designed to help diagnose benign prostatic hyperplasia, it has become clear lately that the quantification of prostatism, although helpful, cannot be used to diagnose benign prostatic hyperplasia, even when the score is elevated because other conditions mentioned above may cause the prostatism symptoms. So this BPH Index needs to be used in the context of evaluating the patient in terms of medical history and possibly other procedures.

The questionnaire consists of seven questions designed to quantify the following symptoms:

1. Urine present in the bladder after urination

2. Urinary frequency

3. Urinary hesitancy

4. Urinary urgency

5. Weakness of urinary stream

6. Difficulty in beginning urination

7. Nocturia (number of nighttime urinations)

Each question is given a score and these are added together for a total score. The total score is then further classified as mild, moderate or severe prostatism. Readers interested in looking at the questionnaire should consult the original article which is available in most medical libraries. See references on page 21.

Digital Rectal Examination (DRE)
The digital rectal examination is less reliable than the symptom survey with regard to diagnosing BPH. Since the part of the prostate that impinges upon the urethra and causes BPH symptoms is the transitional zone surrounding the prostatic urethra deep within the prostate, it cannot be felt on DRE. Although not particularly useful in diagnosing BPH, the DRE is more useful in picking up prostate cancer and in diagnosing prostatitis.

Urinary-Flow Rate Measurement

An important objective method for diagnosing and evaluating BPH is to measure the urinary-flow rate with an electronic instrument called a urinary flow meter. The velocity of urine expelled during urination is the single best test for assessing obstruction of the bladder outlet. The peak flow rate (the rate of urinary flow when the urine is flowing fastest) is a more specific indicator of BPH than the mean rate (the average rate of urinary flow). The rate decreases in all men with advancing age.

When the symptom information obtained from the American Urological Association Symptom Index score is combined with measurements of the urinary-flow rate, the physician can determine the severity of BPH. When a series of these measurements are taken, one has an objective way of evaluating the effectiveness of therapy.

Prostate Specific Antigen (PSA)

PSA is a protein produced by both benign and malignant prostate cells, which can be measured by a simple blood test. It may be abnormally elevated in prostatitis, BPH and prostate cancer. The highest values are generally found in advanced prostate cancer, but one occasionally sees very high values as a result of vigorous stimulation of the prostate, as might occur in a long bike ride. Most physicians consider that its greatest value is in helping to pick up early prostate cancer and to monitor the results of treatment for this condition.

Generally, the guidelines are that a PSA of 0–4 nanograms is considered normal. A PSA over 10 is thought to be high and suggests further evaluation for prostate cancer. Results between 4 and 10 are most likely to be associated with BPH or prostatitis, although prostate cancer is sometimes found at these values or even at normal values of PSA. PSA levels are known to be age-dependent, and deviation from the average range for one's age group may represent a normal deviation and may or may not be indicative of disease.

The Dynamic Component of BPH

The previous discussion has focused on the role of transitional zone enlargement in BPH. However, this is only one component, the so-called static or prostatic enlargement component. A second component is the dynamic component, which reflects the tone or degree of contraction of smooth muscle within the sphincters of the bladder and prostate. When these muscles are stiff or do not relax easily, one can expect urinary flow to be impeded. Current conventional treatment utilizes knowledge of both of these components for the treatment of BPH.

Another possible aspect of the second dynamic component that is generally not mentioned in current American urology textbooks was suggested to me by a European urologist, George Debled, who presented his ideas in a series of lectures in the United States sponsored by the Broda Barnes Foundation of Trumbull, Connecticut. He asserted that the smooth muscles of the prostate were actively involved in helping the urethra to dilate during urination or ejaculation. Thus, although the muscles of the prostate that were involved in sphincter activity needed to relax during urination, the majority of the muscles of the prostate helped the urethra to dilate by contracting appropriately. This notion that smooth muscle activity in the prostate plays a role in promoting urinary flow is extremely important and has major treatment implications for BPH.

Causes of BPH

The exact cause of BPH is unknown. It occurs as men get older, but only when dihydrotestosterone (DHT) is present. The most prevalent current hypothesis for the development of BPH in urology texts and complementary literature is that it is due to an excess of DHT in the prostate. Both conventional and complementary treatments have focused on reducing DHT levels by inhibiting the 5-alpha reductase enzyme. Although DHT does seem to be elevated in BPH tissue in some studies, stopping its production may not be the only way or even the best way of treating BPH. Other approaches will be discussed.

Conventional Surgical Treatment for BPH

An excellent review of the conventional treatments for BPH by Joseph E. Oesterling, M.D., was recently published in the *New England Journal of Medicine*.[2] Until recently, the main conventional treatment for BPH was surgical. If a man had mild BPH symptoms, he was told that the condition was caused by aging and that nothing could be done about it until the symptoms were bad enough. Then, a surgical procedure (removing a portion of the prostate) could be performed which would relieve the symptoms.

According to Oesterling, this approach may not be that unreasonable. "Although intervention may be appropriate for many men with prostatism, doing nothing may be the better management. On the basis of five studies of the natural history of prostatism among men with moderate prostatism who were followed for five years, approximately 40 percent will improve, 45 percent will have no change in symptoms and only 15 percent will have deterioration. . . . Watchful waiting must be considered a management option for men with prostatism." Nevertheless, in recent years, sparked by technological advances and the development of new drugs, many treatment approaches have been developed.

Transurethral Resection of the Prostate (TURP). TURP is a surgical procedure during which the urologist, using an instrument known as a resectoscope, enters the penis through the urethra and snips off prostate tissue that is impinging on the prostatic urethra. This procedure relieves pressure on the urethra, which had been squeezed by the hyperplastic growth of the gland surrounding it. An attempt is made to leave as much healthy tissue as possible and to leave the outer capsule of the prostate gland intact.

Of the treatments to be discussed, the TURP results in the most improvements in symptoms and urinary-flow rate. Long-term followup reveals that more than 75 percent of men undergoing this procedure are satisfied and have good ability to urinate.[3]

Although TURP is an effective treatment for most men with symptomatic BPH, there are considerable problems. Approximately 20 to 25 percent of patients who undergo the procedure do not have satisfactory long-term outcomes.[4] The complications include (1) retrograde ejaculation (the semen is discharged backward into the bladder) in 70 to 75 percent of men; (2) sexual impotence in 5 to 10 percent; (3) postoperative urinary tract infections in 5 to 10 percent; (4) some degree of urinary incontinence in 2 to 4 percent; and (5) a blood transfusion with its risk of infection in 5 to 10 percent. Reoperation is necessary in 15 to 20 percent of men followed for 10 years or more.

Oesterling outlines four minimally invasive methods of treatment for BPH. They are: (1) transurethral incision of the prostate, (2) prostatic stents, (3) microwave therapy, and (4) laser prostatectomy. The first method is available for clinical use in the United States. Prostatic stents, microwave therapy and laser prostatectomy are being studied experimentally in the United States and abroad but are not yet approved by the FDA for treatment for BPH in the United States.

Transurethral Incision of the Prostate (TUIP). This procedure, performed under regional or general anesthesia, is ideal for a patient with a mildly enlarged prostate whose primary obstruction is located at the bladder neck. Either one or two incisions are made across the bladder neck and prostatic urethra. As the incisions are deepened, the bladder neck and prostatic urethra spring open, and the bladder outlet obstruction is relieved. In four prospective, randomized trials comparing TUIP with TURP, TURP showed slightly better results with regard to symptom decrease, but the complication rates were much lower for TUIP. In addition, surgery, hospitalization and convalescence all required a shorter time.

Oesterling concludes: "Transurethral incision of the prostate is ideal not only for men with a small prostate gland, but also for those in whom the preservation of potency and capacity for normal ejaculation are important considerations as well as for debilitated men in whom the risks presented by surgery and anesthesia are substantial. The procedure is markedly underused to treat men with symptomatic benign prostatic hyperplasia."[5]

Conventional Pharmacologic Treatment for BPH

Finasteride (Proscar). The drug Proscar is a potent inhibitor of the enzyme 5-alpha reductase. It is approved by the FDA for the treatment of BPH. The initial studies of finasteride showed that when 5 mg was given orally each day, prostate volume decreased 18 percent, the symptom score decreased 26 percent and the peak urinary-flow rate increased 23 percent.[6] Finasteride acts on the static component of BPH.

A three-year report on the safety and efficacy of finasteride was recently published.[7] Improvements were modest when compared to changes seen with other treatments. Five percent of men treated developed decreased libido, ejaculatory dysfunction or impotence as compared to 1.5 percent of the placebo group. Since finasteride blocks the formation of DHT, it is not surprising to find a rather stark warning in the package insert. It states that the drug has a potential risk for a pregnant woman carrying a male fetus. Apparently, the drug is so lethal that a pregnant woman is warned not to handle Proscar. In addition, if the female sex partner of the patient is to become pregnant, the patient should either discontinue the Proscar or avoid exposure of his semen to his partner. Yet, even with the serious containdications of the drug, a fierce media campaign is being waged to promote Proscar.

Although finasteride is a potent 5-alpha reductase inhibitor and causes a marked decrease in serum and tissue concentrations of DHT, it is only moderately effective in treating symptomatic BPH. For many men the clinical improvement is minimal. Perhaps the most attractive feature is its fairly good toxicity profile, compared to some of the more drastic procedures previously described.

Although suggestions have been made that finasteride may be helpful in preventing prostate cancer, I believe that this is highly unlikely. In fact, the opposite may be true.

Testosterone may be converted either to DHT by the enzyme 5-alpha reductase or to estradiol, the major female sex hormone, by the enzyme aromatase. Considerable evidence exists concerning the role of estrogen and estrogen-like substances in promoting cancer development. If 5-alpha reductase is blocked, one would expect an increase in the estrogen to androgen ratio in the prostate with a resultant increased cancer risk. Time will tell whether blocking 5-alpha reductase results in an increase or decrease in cancer.

Terazosin (Hytrin). By relaxing urinary sphincter spasm (the dynamic component of BPH), the long-acting drug terazosin, whose brand name is Hytrin, as well as other adrenergic agonists, are moderately effective in reducing BPH symptom scores and increasing peak urinary-flow rates. Their onset of action is rapid, and they may also be effective in mild to moderate hypertension. Because these drugs may cause drops in blood pressure on standing, dizziness, headaches and lightheadedness, patients receiving them should be monitored closely. Terazosin did not adversely affect sexual function or alter the PSA, according to recent studies.

PROSTATITIS

Prostatitis is an inflammation of the prostate. The most characteristic symptom of prostatitis, which may not be present in either BPH or prostate cancer, is pain in the prostate or nearby areas. Prostatitis is a condition common among adult men; it is rarely seen in young boys prior to the onset of puberty.

There are four main types of prostatitis.[8] Their names and relative frequencies are: (1) acute and (2) chronic bacterial prostatitis, which constitutes less than 5 percent, (3) nonbacterial prostatitis (64 percent), and prostadynia (31 percent).

Acute Bacterial Prostatitis

Acute bacterial prostatitis is characterized by rapid onset of fever, chills, pain in the lower back and perineum (area between the scrotum and anus) and genitourinary symptoms such as painful and frequent urination, urinary urgency, nocturia, aching muscles, painful joints and general fatigue. Bacteria are found in prostatic secretions and also, most often, in the urine. This condition is particularly common in young, sexually active men.

The diagnosis, based on symptoms and cultures of prostate fluid, is usually easy. Most commonly, the bacterium type causing the condition is *E. coli.* Treatment includes IV and/or oral antibiotics and is usually effective, although occasionally it results in the development of chronic bacterial prostatitis.

Chronic Bacterial Prostatitis

Chronic bacterial prostatitis is characterized by recurrent urinary tract infections caused by the same bacteria type each time, usually *E. coli,* despite repeated courses of antibiotic treatment. Men with this condition may or may not have had acute bacterial prostatitis previously. Most report painful and frequent urination, urgency and nocturia. Prostatic fluid cultures grow out the infecting bacteria.

Response to antibiotic treatment in this condition is not very satisfactory, for the bacterial infection never seems to be completely wiped out and frequently recurs. One reason for this is that antibiotics usually diffuse poorly into the affected tissue, probably because of the extreme alkalinity of the prostate secretions which repel most antibiotics. Somewhat better results are obtained when antibiotics are used for about a month rather than the usual course of ten days.

For those patients who are not cured with the antibiotic treatment, symptoms can usually be suppressed by continuous, suppressive low-dose antibiotics such as Septra.

The prostatic fluid of normal men contains a potent antibacterial factor (PAF) that kills most pathological bacteria that commonly cause genitourinary tract infections. The factor was identified as a zinc compound in 1976. By 1983, Parrish and his colleagues concluded that PAF is free zinc. Since zinc concentrations are low and PAF activity is depressed or absent in the prostatic fluid of men who have chronic bacterial prostatitis, some clinicians believe that zinc (PAF) may serve as a natural defense against ascending genitourinary tract infections in normal men. However, whether the low zinc is a cause of chronic bacterial prostatitis or an effect is not yet totally clear.

Another reason for poor treatment response in chronic bacterial prostatitis is the presence of infected prostatic stones which are fairly common. They can be seen on ultrasound but cannot be detected on rectal examination or on plain X-ray films. Some calculi are made up of constituents commonly found in the urine rather than in prostate secretions, which suggests that components of urine are refluxed into the prostatic ducts to form these calculi. Antibiotics do not appear to eliminate bacteria associated with the stones, and some urologists believe that the only way of dealing with this situation is to remove most of the prostate surgically, thereby removing the stones.

Nonbacterial Prostatitis (NBP)

Nonbacterial prostatitis is the most common type of prostatitis. In this condition, secretions from the prostate are found to contain an abnormally high number of inflammatory cells, as in chronic bacterial prostatitis, but no bacteria are present and no history of any urinary tract infection exists. Symptoms include those of chronic bacterial prostatitis. In addition, a particularly characteristic symptom is postejaculatory pain and discomfort. The cause of nonbacterial prostatitis is unclear. The syndrome may be caused by a yet unidentified microorganism, so it may be a noninfectious disease.

Since the cause of nonbacterial prostatitis is unknown, it is difficult to treat. When the usual bacterial cultures are negative and the physician suspects an organism that does not show up on the usual cultures, a trial of tetracycline or erythromycin may be recommended for about fourteen days. If no improvement takes place, antibiotics should be discontinued. If the patient does improve, a longer course of therapy may be undertaken.

Aside from the rare case that responds to antibiotics, patients with nonbacterial prostatitis are basically told to learn to live with the condition. In some cases, abstaining from alcohol and spicy foods may be helpful. Sitz baths may reduce pain and inflammation. Prostatic massage, which aids in the expulsion of fluid from the congested prostate, may be used, especially in men whose prostate may be congested due to lack of sexual activity. At times anti-inflammatory drugs may relieve symptoms and anti-cholinergic drugs may reduce irritative voiding symptoms. However, since the conventional treatment results of nonbacterial prostatitis are unsatisfactory, the alternative therapies (see page 21) are certainly worth trying.

Prostatodynia (PD)

Prostatodynia is similar to NBP, except that prostatic secretions are normal. That is, the excessive inflammatory cells seen in NBP are not present. Generally, this form of prostatitis occurs in young to middle-aged individuals. The most common and specific symptom is pain and/or discomfort in the groin, perineum, testicles, lower back and penis. Other variable genitourinary symptoms similar to those of NBP may also be experienced.

Patients with prostatodynia have spastic dysfunction of the bladder neck and prostatic urethra which can be seen on video-urodynamic studies. This smooth muscle spasm leads to elevated pressures in the prostatic urethra and subsequent intraprostatic and ejaculatory duct reflux of urine. As the urine refluxes into the prostate, a chemical inflammation of the prostate occurs.

Some patients with prostatodynia seem to suffer primarily from muscular tension in the pelvis floor. Pelvic pain and discomfort are associated with sitting, running or other physical activities that lead to fatigue of these muscles.

The typical PD patient experiences a great deal of emotional strife in his life and seems to have considerable psychosocial and psychosexual pathology. Consequently, many clinicians believe that this plays a major role in the development of prostatodynia. However, it is also possible that the illness plays a considerable role in the psychosocial problems.

Drugs that can help relieve spasms of the smooth muscles and the skeletal muscles of the pelvic floor are used to treat prostatodynia. For the smooth muscle spasm, alpha-adrenergic blocking agents have been used, just as they have been employed to treat the dynamic component of BPH. The dosage must be individualized and continued indefinitely, for the symptoms tend to recur if it is stopped. For skeletal muscle spasms of the pelvic floor, a muscle relaxant, such as Valium may be used. Hot sitz baths, prostatic massage and psychotherapy may also be helpful.

REFERENCES

1. Barry, M. J. Fowler, E. J., Jr., O'Leary, M. P., et al. The American Urological Association Symptom Index for benign prostatic hyperplasia. *J Urol* 148: 1992, 1549–57.
2. Oesterling, J. E. Benign prostatic hyperplasia: medical and minimally invasive treatment options. *N Engl J Med* 332(2): January 12, 1995, 99–108.
3. Bruskewitz, R.C., Larsen, E. H., Madsen, P. O., and Dorfliner, T. 3-Year followup of urinary symptoms after transurethral resection of the prostate. *J Urol* 136: 1986, 613–615.
4. Lepor, H., and Rigaud, G. The efficacy of transurethral resection of the prostate in men with moderate symptoms of prostatism. *J Urol* 143: 1990, 533–537.
5. Oesterling, J. E. Benign prostatic hyperplasia: medical and minimally invasive treatment options. *N Engl J Med* 332: 1995, 99–109.
6. Rittmaster, R. S. Finasteride. *N Eng J Med* 330: 1994, 120–125.
7. Stoner, E. Three-year safety and efficacy data on the use of finasteride in the treatment of benign prostatic hyperplasia. *Urology* 43: 1994, 284–294.
8. Meares, E. M., Jr., Prostatitis and related disorders. In *Campbell's Urology*, 6th edition, ed. Walsh, P. C., Retik, A. B., et al., W. B. Saunders Co., Philadelphia, PA, 1992, 807–822.

COMPLEMENTARY PREVENTION AND TREATMENT OF BPH AND PROSTATITIS

Conventional treatments of prostate disorders are centered around symptom relief either by drug treatment or surgical procedures. Conventional medicine pays little attention to the possible role played by diet, lifestyle, natural nonprescriptive substances and environmental factors in causing, preventing or treating prostate problems. The complementary approach to preventing and treating BPH and prostatitis focuses on these areas.

DIETARY RECOMMENDATIONS

The following basic nutritional principles are guidelines for any patient interested in improving his health. Whenever I see a man with a prostate problem or any other medical problem in my practice, I start with general recommendations along with specifics for his particular problem. The specific program has a much better chance of succeeding when these general guidelines are followed. In addition, the general guidelines may require modification to deal with individual biological differences, cultural differences, individual preferences and factors such as food allergies. Nevertheless, most people would benefit by attempting to follow these general principles.

We generally emphasize a high fiber, high complex carbohydrate, relatively low fat and moderate protein diet. This diet is high in fruits, vegetables and whole grains; contains modest amounts of nuts and seeds; modest amounts of animal protein such as organic chicken and fish; and fresh raw vegetable juices, including carrots, greens and apples. We encourage the use of organic foods, whenever possible, and we allow modest amounts of organic eggs and dairy products. Occasionally, we recommend organic red meats for certain metabolic types.

Avoid List

Because some of the items, like caffeine, are addictive and produce withdrawal symptoms when they are removed from the diet suddenly, I often recommend that use of such substances be eliminated slowly.

- **Sugar**
  Avoid all foods containing added refined sugar (e.g., cakes, candies, ice cream, sodas, certain cereals, jello, ketchup). Raw unfiltered honey, unsulphured black strap molasses, pure maple syrup and rice syrup may be used as sweeteners but only in moderation.

- **Alcohol**
  Avoid all alcoholic beverages including liquor, beer and wine. Try naturally sparkling spring water with a twist of lemon or lime as your social drink.

- **Caffeine**
  Avoid coffee, tea, cola and chocolate as well as chemically treated decaffeinated coffee. Water-processed decaffeinated coffee or tea in moderation is fine. Herb teas and health food store "coffee substitutes" such as Pero or Postum are also acceptable.

- **Tobacco**
  Avoid cigarettes, cigars, pipes, and the like. Try to avoid inhaling other people's smoke, as much as possible.

- **White flour products**
  Avoid white bread, including enriched breads, white pasta products, white rice and any processed foods containing white flour. Whole grain flour products and brown rice should be used instead.

- **Hydrogenated fats**
  Avoid hydrogenated and partially hydrogenated fats (e.g., margarine, Crisco and processed peanut butter). Old-fashioned, untreated organic peanut butter, free of aflatoxins, should be used instead of processed peanut butter. Label reading is essential. Saturated fats (e.g., butter, animal fats, coconut products) are allowed in moderation. Unsaturated cold-pressed vegetable oils (e.g., safflower, sesame, canola, sunflower, virgin olive oil) may be used. Avoid deep frying in vegetable oils; for light sautéing, olive oil should be used. Broth may also be used for this purpose.

- **Chemicals added to food**
  Labels must be read. Avoid artificial preservatives (e.g., BHA, BHT, MSG, nitrites, nitrates, sodium benzoates, etc.) commonly found in bread, crackers and cereals. All processed cured meats such as bologna, salami, frankfurters, corned beef and pastrami should be avoided because of the addition of chemicals. Avoid artificial coloring commonly found in frankfurters, soda, candy, maraschino cherries, some juice drinks and so on. Avoid artificial flavoring commonly found in certain ice creams, frozen pies and candy. Avoid artificial sweeteners such as aspartame (Nutrasweet or Equal) and saccharine (Sweet 'n Low). These are found in all diet sodas, diabetic foods and other processed low calorie foods.

- **Fluoride and chlorine**
  Avoid fluoridated water, chlorinated water and all tap water, unless it is appropriately filtered. Use bottled spring water, distilled or filtered water. Although boiling water removes

chlorine, it only concentrates fluoride. To remove fluoride from tap water, a filtering process that includes reverse osmosis is necessary. Check with your water company to find out if your tap water is fluoridated. Avoid fluoridated toothpaste. A variety of brands of toothpaste without fluoride are available at health food stores. However, some brands in health food stores do contain fluoride, so labels must be read carefully.

- **Aluminum and Teflon cookware**
  Aluminum tends to accumulate in the body, and fluoride may be released from Teflon. Use stainless steel, pyrex, enamel, Corning and iron cookware instead.

- **Nonprescription drugs**
  Avoid marijuana, cocaine, hallucinogens (e.g., LSD) and all recreational drugs.

- **Prescription drugs**
  Take prescription drugs only if absolutely necessary. Try to keep these to a minimum.

- **Amalgam (mercury containing) dental fillings**
  Mercury is highly toxic. It enters the tissues of the body and damages the nervous system, immune system and other systems. Ask your dentist for other alternatives.

- **Electric blankets**
  The electric energy field interferes with one's own energy field.

- **Hair dyes**
  Synthetic hair dyes increase risk for certain types of cancers. Some men's hair dyes contain lead. Certain natural, vegetable-derived dyes may be more acceptable.

- **High voltage power lines**
  Avoid these as much as possible, for they have been linked to increased rates of cancer and leukemia in children, and other disorders. If your home is located near them, consider moving.

- **Waterbeds**
  The electric energy field used to warm the bed interferes with one's own energy field.

- **Metal-rimmed eyeglasses**
  The metal crossing the midline between the eyes weakens one's energy field.

NUTRITIONAL SUPPLEMENTS

Several specific natural substances may be used to prevent or treat BPH and prostatitis. These include specific vitamins, minerals, essential fatty acids, specific amino acids and herbs. In taking nutritional supplements it is important to keep in mind that they work as a team to achieve optimal balance in the body. Although all nutrients are useful to some extent, those included here have either shown specific usefulness in prostate disorders or are necessary for balance when the specific prostate nutrients are taken.

Zinc

The single most important nutrient for a healthy prostate is the mineral zinc. Present in small amounts in the human body, zinc, an essential mineral, is involved in healing wounds, bolstering the immune system, protecting the liver from chemical damage, sharpening the senses of taste and smell and forming collagen which, among other things, is a precursor of bone. Many Americans are deficient in zinc because much of our soil has been depleted of this mineral due to modern farming techniques. In addition, the processing of food generally depletes zinc and other minerals and many Americans ingest large amounts of processed food.

The normal prostate gland contains more zinc than any other body organ (up to ten times more). In contrast to normal prostate tissue, prostate cancer cells contain greatly reduced quantities of zinc. This change in prostate cancer cells may precede the anatomical appearance of the prostate cancer cells.

Zinc deficiency has been shown to cause enlargement of the prostate gland. With regard to BPH, zinc is helpful in two specific ways. First, it reduces the level of circulating prolactin by inhibiting prolactin secretion. Prolactin is a hormone that aids in the uptake of testosterone by the prostate. Increased testosterone uptake tends to activate the enzyme 5-alpha reductase, promoting DHT and stimulating prostate growth.

Promotors of increased prolactin levels include beer, psychosocial stress and the amino acid tryptophan. Eliminating beer and reducing stress can thus be beneficial in reducing the BPH process.

The second specific way that zinc is helpful in BPH is that it affects the activity of 5-alpha reductase. Some zinc is necessary for the enzyme to work properly, but higher levels of zinc tend to inhibit 5-alpha reductase activity, thus reducing DHT formation and inhibiting BPH.

Zinc is also helpful to patients with prostatitis. It enhances immune function in general, thus improving the body's ability to fight bacteria and other microorganisms anywhere in the body, including the prostate. Specifically within the prostate gland, PAF, the antibiotic-like substance discussed earlier, has actually been determined to be free zinc, a finding which points to zinc as a natural defense against prostate infections in men.

In using zinc as a supplement one should be aware that it can lead to a deficiency of copper, another trace mineral because copper and zinc compete for absorption. In general, the ratio of zinc to copper supplementation should be between 7:1 and 14:1 in favor of zinc:copper. Thus, if 50 mg of zinc is given, then at least 4 mg of copper should also be prescribed and taken at a different time during the day.

For prostate problems, I recommend zinc picolinate because of its excellent absorption. The dosage of elemental zinc should be between 15 mg and 60 mg daily. An appropriate amount of copper should also be taken as a supplement, preferably at a different time of day from the zinc. The form of copper that I have found to be particularly useful is copper sebacate. Blood, urine or hair levels of zinc may be used to help monitor the proper dosage. In taking zinc, other important considerations are that iron inhibits and vitamin B6 enhances zinc absorption. So, iron should not be taken at the same time as zinc, and vitamin B6 should be part of the supplement program.

Vitamin B6 (Pyridoxine)

Vitamin B6 may be used as a supplement for prostate problems because it enhances the absorption of zinc and it may help to inhibit excessive prolactin production by the pituitary. The dosage may range from 50 to several hundred milligrams of vitamin B6 daily. When using B6, it is wise to add at least modest doses of other B vitamins and some magnesium in the range of 300-800 mg daily.

Magnesium

Magnesium is helpful for benign prostate problems to improve muscle function, aiding appropriate skeletal and smooth muscle relaxation and contraction and aiding the immune system to help deal with prostatitis. It is also necessary to balance high doses of vitamin B6. It may be helpful in preventing calcium stones in the prostrate because of its natural antagonism to calcium. On the other hand, sufficient calcium must either be in the diet or also be given as a supplement. The dosage range for elemental magnesium would be somewhere between 300 and 800 mg daily. I prefer to use magnesium in the glycinate or taurate form.

Amino Acids

Certain amino acids have been found to provide some relief of symptoms. For example, in one study of 45 men taking a combination of the three amino acids glycine, alanine and glutamic acid, 95 percent reported improvement in nocturia, 81 percent in urgency and 73 percent in frequency.[1] Several supplement companies include these three amino acids in their prostate support preparations. Approximate daily doses for these three amino acids are: glutamic acid 1,000 mg; alanine 50 mg; and glycine 400 mg, given in divided doses.

Saw Palmetto

Extracts of the saw palmetto berry (also called *serenoa repens*) are extremely valuable for the management of BPH and to some extent prostatitis. The daily dosage of this extract is 320 mg per day (or two 80 mg capsules given twice daily). Most of the prepared extracts are 30 times more potent than the preparations of dry, powdered, whole berries. In traditional Chinese medicine, the berry has been used in the treatment of many male urogenital disturbances as well as mammary gland disorders. In contrast to Proscar, which tends to reduce libido in some patients, many herbalists regard saw palmetto as a mild aphrodisiac.[2]

With regard to the prostate, saw palmetto is useful in the treatment of BPH as well as prostatitis. Considerable research has been done with saw palmetto both clinically and to determine mechanisms of action in vitro. With regard to BPH, it is a natural inhibitor of 5-alpha reductase.[3] This has the obvious effect of limiting the conversion of testosterone to DHT. It also binds to the androgen protein receptor that must combine with DHT before the complex can have its effect in the nucleus of the cell.[4] This reduces the physiological effects of DHT and results in DHT being broken down and excreted instead of used. For prostatitis, the fat-soluble extract of the berry has anti-inflammatory properties and immune-stimulatory effects.

In his small monograph, entitled *The Saw Palmetto Story*, Michael Murray, N.D., outlines the results of eleven clinical studies demonstrating the effectiveness of *serenoa repens* in BPH. Six of these studies were double-blind, placebo-controlled studies, and five were open studies. All of them showed significant positive results. Among the variables checked in one or more studies were: volume voided, maximum flow, mean flow, dysuria, nocturia, number of voidings, residual urine and other BPH symptoms.[5] No significant side effects have ever been reported from the use of saw palmetto, as far as I have been able to determine.

In a Merck-sponsored study, cited by Whitaker,[6] comparing Proscar with saw palmetto, Proscar was shown to be a stronger inhibitor of 5-alpha reductase than saw palmetto in an in-vitro study. Proscar was also able to reduce blood DHT more than saw palmetto. However, saw palmetto appeared to be superior to Proscar with regard to clinical effects when comparing the change of urine-flow rate between a group of pooled patients on saw palmetto and a group on Proscar. At the end of three months, the Proscar group showed a 16 percent improvement while the saw palmetto group improved 38 percent.

Saw palmetto extract has been used in France since 1982 where it is marketed as Permixon. In the United States it has not yet received FDA approval for the treatment of BPH or prostatitis. However, the extract is sold here in health food stores, either alone or in combination with other substances useful for the prostate.

Pygeum Africanum and Stinging Nettles

Pygeum africanum is an evergreen tree that grows about 100 feet tall in central and southern Africa. Native tribes were the first to use the bark of this tree to treat genitourinary symptoms. The bark contains anti-inflammatory and antibacterial substances, as well as substances that help to reduce cholesterol levels in the body. Excessive cholesterol levels are associated with increased prostate cellular growth.

Pygeum africanum has been used to treat prostate disorders in Europe since the early 1980s. Approximately 80 percent of the prescriptions for BPH in France include this herb. Several European double-blind, placebo-controlled studies attest to its efficacy. Translations of abstracts of these studies may be found in a report by Dr. James Balch.[7] One French study involved two random groups of sixty patients who were given either an extract of *Pygeum africanum* or a placebo. The *Pygeum* group showed a statistically significant reduction in number of urinations per night, ease in starting urination and a more complete emptying of the bladder. A 60 day, randomized, Italian study of 40 patients with nonadvanced BPH showed that the group receiving 100 milligrams of a standardized *Pygeum africanum* extract had statistically significant improvement compared to the placebo group in urinary frequency, urinary urgency, painful urination and urine flow in the patients treated with the active substance.

A much larger multicenter, randomized, double-blind, placebo-controlled German study involved 263 patients and was carried out in eight centers in Germany, France and Austria. Capsules containing either 50 milligrams of *Pygeum africanum* extract or placebo were given twice daily for 60 days. Overall assessment at the end of therapy showed that urination improved in 66 percent of the patients treated with *Pygeum africanum* extract and 31 percent of the placebo group. The only observed side effects were gastrointestinal symptoms, which occurred in five patients, requiring discontinuation of treatment in three of them.

Individual herbs are often more effective when used in combination with other herbs. This was the case in a study which combined *Pygeum africanum* with stinging nettles (*urtica dioica*), a common herb that is often used for nasal allergies. In a randomized double-blind, placebo-controlled study of 63 patients comparing the efficacy of treating BPH with *Pygeum africanum* alone versus a combination of *Pygeum afri-*

canum and stinging nettles, the combination was superior in improving urinary flow and reducing residual urine. The dosage was one capsule twice daily of 300 mg of a standardized extract of the roots of stinging nettles (concentrated at a ratio of 5:1) and 25 mg of a standardized extract of the bark of *Pygeum africanum*, using a recently introduced, highly concentrated extract of 200:1.[8]

Unpublished data from studies of the mechanism of action of the nettle/Pygeum extract indicate that its principal effects are based on the inhibition of 5-alpha reductase. Pygeum is a potent inhibitor, whereas nettle is somewhat weaker. Both extracts also inhibit aromatase, the enzyme that converts testosterone to estradiol. Both of these actions tend to improve BPH.[9]

Pygeum africanum is most commonly taken in pill form for several months. In addition to being combined with stinging nettles, Pygeum may also be combined with saw palmetto.

Flower Pollen

Pollen has shown beneficial results in the prevention and treatment of prostate disorders. It overflows with beneficial nutrients including the B vitamins, vitamin E, amino acids, fatty acids, carotenoids and minerals.

A European flower pollen product called Cernilton has shown effectiveness in the treatment of both BPH symptoms and prostatitis.[10] Flower or bee pollen has been shown to relax the sphincter muscle of the bladder, thus reducing symptoms of urinary obstruction. Double-blind crossover studies have confirmed the beneficial effects of flower pollen in BPH and prostatitis.[11,12] The usual dosage of Cernilton flower pollen is about six capsules daily. Some components of pollen block free radicals and stimulate the immune system. Anti-inflammatory activities are present. Bee pollen has also been used for prostate problems, but supporters of the use of flower pollen argue that flower pollen is superior.

Essential Fatty Acids

Like vitamins, essential fatty acids must be ingested from the diet; they cannot be manufactured by the body. There are two classes of essential fatty acids: the omega-3 series and the omega-6 series. Alpha linolenic acid, found in high concentrations in flax oil, represents the omega-3 series, while gamma linolenic acid, or GLA, found in evening primrose oil, is a good representative of the omega-6 series. Both of these fatty acids are capable of making local hormones called prostaglandins that have anti-inflammatory and anticancer properties. To treat BPH and prostatitis, one member of each class should be used. I usually recommend one to two tablespoons of flaxseed oil and 6 to 12 capsules of evening primrose oil daily. Whenever essential fatty acids are taken, it is important to increase one's intake of vitamin E and selenium. Along with these oils, I recommend about 800 units of vitamin E, as mixed tocopherols, and 200 to 400 mcg of selenium as sodium selenite.

Suggested Nutrients for BPH and Prostatitis

Supplement	Daily Amount
Zinc picolinate	15–60 mg
Vitamin B$_6$	50–300 mg
Magnesium glycinate or taurate	200–600 mg of elemental magnesium
Saw palmetto (80 mg each)	2 capsules 2x daily
Pygeum africanum (*200:1 concentrate*)	25–50 mg
Stinging nettle leaves (*5:1 concentrate*)	150–300 mg
Cernilton flower pollen	6 capsules
Flaxseed oil	1–2 Tbs. or 12 caps
Evening primrose oil (500 mg each)	6–12 caps
Vitamin E (400 I.U. each)	1 cap 2x daily
Sodium selenite	200–400 mcg of elemental selenium
Copper sebacate	4 mg of elemental copper
Amino acids (*glycine, alanine and glutamic acid*)	6 caps
Multi vitamin/mineral	

The above program should be helpful for most patients with BPH or prostatitis. For most patients, a combination of only a few of these supplements is all that is necessary. To help pinpoint which would be most beneficial may require the help of a complementary physician or might be established through trial and error.

On the other hand, many other nutrients might also be helpful. For example, immune-enhancing antioxidants such as vitamin C, vitamin A and beta carotene might be added to the program. All of these supplements should be used in the context of the dietary recommendations and the "avoid list" mentioned earlier.

TESTOSTERONE THERAPY

The predominant hypothesis for the development of BPH is the buildup of DHT within the prostate which promotes prostate growth. The primary pharmacologic treatment has been the use of 5-alpha reductase inhibitors to reduce the formation of DHT. But can DHT buildup really be the cause of BPH? Although some studies indicate an increase in DHT in the prostate cells of BPH patients compared to normal prostates of patients the same age, the blood levels of both testosterone and DHT levels generally decline with age. Younger men generally have higher levels of testosterone and DHT, but do not have BPH.

The presence of DHT in prostate cells is necessary for prostate enlargement, so it follows that a reduction of DHT would tend to reduce the size of the prostate. But just because DHT must be present for the prostate to enlarge in size, it does not necessarily follow that the best approach to reducing the size of the prostate or preventing BPH is to eliminate or drastically reduce DHT production.

In order for BPH to occur, a man must be older and have DHT present in his prostate. The hormonal changes that occur in an aging man relate more to an increase in other hormones such as estradiol, a female sex hormone, prolactin from the pituitary, and LH and FSH from the pituitary which are associated with falling testosterone and DHT blood levels. Among all androgen-metabolizing enzymes within the human prostate, 5-alpha reductase is the most powerful one. The activity of this enzyme in younger men is much higher in the glandular cells than in the muscle and connective tissue cells. However, with aging, its activity in the glandular cells *decreases,* while in the muscle and connective tissue, it remains constant over the whole age range. Thus, in older prostates with BPH, the activity is almost the same in both compartments.

In contrast to DHT, estrogens are increasingly accumulated in the muscles and connective tissue of the prostate with advancing age, whereas in the glandular cells, the estrogen level remains constant over the whole age range. The age-dependent decrease of the DHT level in the glandular cells and the increase in estrogen in the muscle and connective tissue cells lead to a significant increase of the estrogen/androgen ratio. This could be of pathobiological importance for BPH development.[13]

The Male Andropause

George Debled, M.D., a European urologist, suggests that testosterone deficiency rather than excess DHT is important in the development of BPH and prostatitis. Since the mid-1970s, he has run a clinic for men which specializes in sexual dysfunction and prostate problems. During this time, he has successfully treated approximately 2,000 patients. For these patients, Dr. Debled generally orders a male hormone blood profile consisting of (1) Total Serum Testosterone, (2) Free Serum Testosterone, (3) Serum DHT, (4) Serum FSH, (5) Serum LH, (6) Estradiol, (7) Estrone and (8) Sex Hormone Binding Globulin. He has found that young men with impotency or libido problems often have sex hormone blood levels similar to those of older men with prostate problems. That is, testosterone and especially free testosterone levels are reduced, and FSH, LH, estradiol, estrone and sex hormone binding globulin levels are increased. As a result of these hormonal changes, men in their forties, fifties and sixties develop slow changes in their bodies analogous to women going through menopause. This phenomenon has been termed the male climacteric, or *an-*

dropause. Treating these patients with testosterone generally improves their sexual functioning, including libido and potency problems. In addition, testosterone positively impacts the prostate gland.

Nourishing the Prostate Gland with Testosterone

Dr. Debled points out that testosterone is necessary to nourish all of the tissues of the male urinary and reproductive systems, including the prostate. Testosterone nurtures the development of muscles and is necessary for proper muscular functioning. When the muscle tissue of the bladder and the prostate does not receive sufficient testosterone, it tends to function poorly, atrophy and fibrose. This may then help to explain some of the symptoms involving bladder irritability which are not well explained by an obstructive hypothesis. If the smooth muscle in the prostate does not function properly, the prostatic urethra will not dilate properly, resulting in an impaired dynamic component of urination and an impaired urinary flow. The abstract of a recent European paper on BPH reveals that not all symptoms of BPH are due to obstruction. In a significant proportion of patients admitted for TURP, no obstruction is present in over one-fourth of patients.[14]

A cessation of all testosterone production will cause a complete atrophy or shrinkage and loss of function of the prostate. So although a testosterone deficiency may result in a reduction in size of the prostate, prostate function will be impaired and poor urinary function may develop in spite of the reduced size.

Rather than trying to inhibit the formation of DHT, Debled administers testosterone to patients with symptoms of sexual dysfunction, prostate symptoms and low testosterone levels. He believes that he can reduce the symptoms of BPH and prostatitis and forestall BPH surgical procedures for at least 10 years by giving men testosterone. His treatment does not include lifestyle changes, nutritional supplements, herbs and other complementary treatments that have been discussed here. The addition of these therapeutic modalities might further improve his results.

Other Benefits of Testosterone Therapy

According to Dr. Debled and a number of studies involving testosterone, the therapeutic benefits of testosterone therapy go far beyond its effects on the reproductive and urinary system. In addition to its effects on male sexuality and secondary sex characteristics, testosterone improves general motivation and drive. It also has profound effects on other more generalized metabolic functions, including positive effects on the heart and cardiovascular system, blood sugar, bone density, muscle mass and the immune system[15].

Administration of Testosterone

Natural testosterone may be administered by several routes, including oral micronized capsules, a cream applied to the scrotum, a patch applied to the scrotum, sublingual lozenges or intramuscular injections—either short-acting or long-acting. Some of these forms are available only from compounding pharmacies.

Many synthetic testosterone derivatives such as methyl testosterone are approved by the FDA; however, I believe these synthetics should be avoided. Methyl testosterone may cause liver damage and even liver cancer. It has been removed from the market in several European countries. The intramuscular injectable forms consist of testosterone combined with an acid such as proprionic acid or cypionic acid. These forms appear to be reasonably safe. All of the other forms that I recommend are pure natural testosterone.

BALANCING OTHER HORMONES

For optimal prostate functioning, all of the endocrine glands need to be in balance. Consequently, a full evaluation would include checks on the thyroid, adrenals and the pituitary. Imbalances might be corrected by the judicious use of other natural hormones, such as desiccated thyroid or the adrenal hormone, dehydroepiandrosterone (DHEA).

Exercise

No complementary program for the prostate would be complete without mentioning the important role of exercise. Walking is one of the best exercises for helping to keep the prostate healthy. A minimum of 30 minutes daily should be spent in a moderate exercise program such as walking.

To improve urinary control, men may practice so-called Kegel exercises, which involve contracting the muscles of the pelvic floor. This can be done by contracting the muscles as if you were trying to stop a bowel movement or urinary flow. These brief contractions can be built up to a hundred or more times daily if there is any evidence of loss of urinary control.

Stretching exercises, as practiced in hatha yoga or a similar discipline, can improve circulation and flexibility and also contribute to a healthy prostate.

Sexual Activity

A moderate degree of regular sexual activity helps to keep the prostate healthy. Frequent and intense sexual stimulation without orgasm and ejaculation may tend to irritate the prostate and contribute to prostatitis. On the other hand, very little sexual activity may also result in problems. Low libido and other sexual dysfunctions may be helped by many of the measures that have previously been discussed, including correcting testosterone deficiencies.

Stress Management

Emotional and psychological stress can cause imbalances in the autonomic nervous system and contribute to prostate problems, especially prostatodynia. A variety of stress management procedures may be helpful. These may include psychotherapy, meditation practices, hatha yoga, relaxation exercises, autogenic training, deep breathing exercises and many others. Sufficient rest and sleep are also important to keep stress levels manageable. Fresh air and exposure to indirect sunlight through the eyes are important to balance both the immune system and the endocrine system.

REFERENCES

1. Feinblatt, H. M. Palliative treatment of BPH: value of glycine, alanine, glutamic acid combination. *J Maine Med Assoc* 49:99, 1958.
2. Pizzorno, J. E., and Murray, M. T. *A Textbook of Natural Medicine. Chapter 5-Serenoa Repens.* JBC Publications, Seattle, WA, 1989.
3. Sultan, C., Terraza, A., Devillier, C., Carilla, E., Briley, M., Loire, C., and Descomps, B. Inhibition of androgen metabolism and binding by a liposterolic extract of Serenoa Repens B in human foreskin fibroblasts. *J. Steroid Biochem* 20: 1984, 515–519.
4. Briley, M., Carilla, E., and Fauran, F. Permixon, a new treatment for benign prostatic hyperplasia, acts directly at the cytosolic androgen receptor in the rat prostate. *Br. J. Pharmac* 79: 1983, 327.
5. Murray, M. *The Saw Palmetto Story: The Health Series.* Vital Communications, 1990.
6. Whitaker, J. *The Prostate Report: Prevention and Healing.* Phillips Publishing, Potomac, MD, 1994.
7. Balch, J. *Prostate Health.* Alternative Medicine Updates, Marine del Rey, CA, 1994.
8. Montaneri, E., Mandressi, A., Magri, V., et al. Phytotherapy of benign prostatic hypertrophy (BPH) without complications. *Der informierte Arzt* 6A: 1991, 593–598.
9. Krezeski, T., Kazon, M., Borkowski, A., Witeska, A., and Kuczera, J. Combined extracts of *urtica dioica* and *pygeum africanum* in the treatment of benign prostatic hyperplasia: double-blind comparison of two doses. *Clinical Therapeutics* 15(6): 1993, 1012.
10. Leander, G. A preliminary investigation on the therapeutic effects of Cernilton in chronic prosatovesiculitis. *Svenska Lak. Tidn.*, 59: 1962, 3296.
11. Ask-Upmark, E. Prostatitis and its treatment. *Acta Med Scand.*, 181: 1967, 355–357.
12. Inada, T., Kiragawa, T., and Miyakawa, M. Use of Cernilton in patients with prostatic hypertrophy. *Acta urol* (Kyoto) 13: 1967, 466.

13. Krieg, M., Weisser, H., and Tunn, S. Androgen and estrogen metabolism in human benign prostatic hyperplasia (BPH). *Verh-Dtsch-Ges-Pathol*, 77: 1993, 19–24.
14. Schafer, W., Urodynamics in benign prostatic hyperplasia (BPH). *Arch-Ital-Urol-Androl*, 65(6): 1993, 599–613.
15. Moller, J. *Cholesterol: Interactions with Testosterone and Cortisol in Cardiovascular Diseases.* Springer-Verlag, Berlin, Heidelberg, Germany, 1987.

PROSTATE CANCER

According to the American Cancer Society, in 1995 one out of six American men will be diagnosed with prostate cancer; an estimated 244,000 men will be diagnosed with the disease and 40,400 will die from it. Overall, it is the most common malignancy in American men, recently exceeding even lung cancer. In men over age 55, it is the second most common cause of death due to cancer. At autopsy, approximately 10 to 30 percent of men over the age of 50 are found to have some malignant prostate cells, even if the diagnosis of cancer was never made during life.[1] A recent study indicates that this figure may be even higher in relatively young men.[2] In men over the age of 90, the rate approaches 100 percent. The prostate cancers not recognized during the life of the patient are referred to as histologic carcinomas, since they are recognized by a pathologist as looking cancerous but do not cause their host any signs or symptoms of cancer.[3] At least 95 percent of all prostate cancer is of a type called adenocarcinoma, which means that it arises in the glandular cells of the prostate.

The incidence of prostate cancer varies with geographical location. The worldwide incidence of prostate cancer is highest among African Americans and lowest among Asians. In the United States, there are 14 prostate cancer-related deaths per 100,000 men each year. In Sweden, the number is 22 per 100,000 and in Japan, only 2. However, when Japanese men migrate to the United States, their prostate cancer-related death rate approaches that of American men, suggesting that environment, especially diet, plays a major role in the development of clinical prostate cancer.

SYMPTOMS AND SIGNS

Some of the symptoms and signs of prostate cancer are similar to those of prostatitis or BPH. They may include pain on urination, difficulty voiding or a narrowed stream, an increased frequency of urination, urinary retention or blood in the urine. If the cancer has already spread to the bones, then back, hip or other bony pain may be present. Of course, in advanced undiagnosed cases, one may see generalized cancer symptoms, such as loss of appetite, weight loss, general malaise and fatigue. However, many cases of prostate cancer exhibit no symptoms whatsoever at the time of diagnosis.

EVALUATING AND DIAGNOSING PROSTATE CANCER

Since early prostate cancer is frequently asymptomatic, we need some tools to help us make an early diagnosis. Fortunately, three relatively noninvasive methods are available to help screen for prostate cancer. They are (1) the digital rectal examination, which is done during a complete physical examination, (2) a blood test known as prostatic specific antigen (PSA), and (3) a transrectal ultrasound examination of the prostate.

Digital Rectal Exam (DRE)
Until a few years ago, the main diagnostic screening test for prostate cancer was the digital rectal examination (DRE). Prostate cancer is suggested when the examining physician palpates one or more stony hard nodules on the prostate.

However, many prostate cancers are not felt during this examination. Nevertheless, the American Cancer Society recommends that asymptomatic men over the age of 40 be screened for prostate cancer annually with a DRE.

Prostatic Specific Antigen (PSA)
The major recent change in the diagnosis of prostate cancer is the use of the PSA blood test as a screening tool for prostate cancer. PSA is a protein produced by both benign and malignant cells. It can be abnormally elevated in prostatitis and BPH as well as in prostate cancer. Since both false positive and false negative results may occur, it cannot be regarded as a definitive test for prostate cancer. When it is above 20, the most likely diagnosis is prostate cancer that has spread beyond the prostate capsule. Between 10 and 20, the diagnosis may be either prostate cancer, BPH or prostatitis, but it most likely is prostate cancer. Between 5 and 10, the diagnosis is most likely BPH, but prostate cancer could be present. In fact, 25 percent of biopsy-proven, early-stage prostate cancers have a normal PSA. Nevertheless, the PSA as a screening test for prostate cancer is approximately 50 percent more sensitive than a digital rectal examination.

Currently, there is a national debate regarding whether the easy-to-use PSA screening technique is a blessing or a curse. Some believe the test is not sensitive or specific enough to use as a population-wide screening device. There is a fear that the high proportion of false positive results will lead to an "epidemic of treatment." The treatment epidemic would include people who have (1) an elevated PSA for a reason other than cancer and (2) an asymptomatic, either slow-growing or latent cancer and who probably would have died from some other cause before they ever noticed they had cancer. These people would be urged to undergo unnecessary and potentially debilitating surgery.

At this time, a national screening program for prostate cancer using PSA is taking place, in spite of the views of its opponents. Many experts suggest that men over the age of 50 receive both a DRE and PSA each year to screen for prostate cancer.

Transrectal Ultrasound of the Prostate (TRUS-P)

One method of evaluating the prostate is to get an image or a picture of it. Transrectal ultrasound of the prostate or TRUS-P involves inserting an ultrasound probe into the rectum and obtaining images of the prostate and surrounding structures. From these images, a fairly accurate estimate of the size of the prostate can be made, and abnormal nodules suggestive of prostate cancer can be seen.

Ultrasound may also be used to guide a needle during a needle biopsy. The advent of TRUS-P has increased early-detection capabilities. In one study, the procedure detected cancer in 50 percent of individuals who had previously had a negative biopsy performed by palpation (non-needle-guided).[4] A TRUS-P is usually done if a PSA level is elevated or if the digital rectal examination (DRE) is positive. When the DRE and PSA are normal, a transrectal ultrasound of the prostate study is unlikely to enhance the rate of detection of prostate cancer.

In addition to helping determine the presence of cancer, the TRUS-P is helpful in staging the cancer, once it has been diagnosed. This is done by supplying information about the size and degree of spread of a tumor. One advantage of the transrectal ultrasound of the prostate compared to X rays or CT scans is that exposure to ultrasound waves appears to be less dangerous than exposure to ionizing radiation which occurs with X rays and CT scans.

Biopsy

The only conclusive means of determining the presence and type of prostate cancer is a positive biopsy. This is unfortunate because the procedure itself is somewhat risky, especially the danger of spreading a cancer through cutting it or via a needle biopsy. A biopsy involves removing a tissue sample from the prostate for review by a pathologist. The criteria for doing a prostate biopsy include (1) the palpation of a nodule on DRE, (2) a PSA level above 10 ng/ml, and (3) a positive finding on TRUS-P often done when the PSA is between 4 and 10 ng/ml.

STAGING AND GRADING

Once prostate cancer is diagnosed, knowledge of its stage is essential to carry out a conventional treatment plan. *Staging* the prostate cancer refers to the location and extent of the cancer, while *grading* refers to the appearance of cancer cells under the microscope.

The stages of prostate cancer are divided into four major stages, namely, A, B, C and D. Stages A, B and C represent localized disease, whereas stage D indicates that the prostate cancer has spread outside the local area to regional lymph nodes or distantly to the lungs or bones. Stage A represents the earliest and most successfully treatable stage, whereas stage D reflects the most advanced and least treatable stage.

The diagnosis of stage A occurs when the pathological specimen from an operation for BPH shows microscopic evidence of malignancy. In stage B the prostate cancer is confined to the prostate gland as it is in stage A, but a nodule may be felt on digital rectal examination. Stage C prostate cancer manifests as a large mass involving all or most of the prostate gland and is not confined to the gland. With stage D, we have evidence of metastatic prostate cancer.

In contrast to the staging system of prostate cancer which focuses mostly on the location of the cancer, the grading system focuses on the appearance of the cancer under the microscope. The shape, size and arrangement of the cancer cells in the prostate gland reflect the aggressiveness of the cancer. Well-differentiated cancer cells look most like normal tissue, and such cancers usually have the most benign course. The most poorly differentiated consists of irregular masses that have invaded connective tissue. These cancers exhibit the worst prognosis. The Gleason system is often used to quantify the grade of a prostate cancer histological specimen. In general, 2 to 4 is considered well differentiated, 5 to 7 moderately well differentiated and 8 to 10 poorly differentiated.

OTHER DIAGNOSTIC PROCEDURES

From a conventional point of view, treatment options are strongly linked to the stage of the prostate cancer. Therefore, it is crucial to determine the stage of the disease prior to commencing treatment. Unfortunately, in spite of all the technology available to us, the stage of the disease is often underestimated, resulting in needless mutilating and dangerous procedures. The major question is whether or not the cancer is confined to the prostate gland or whether the cancer has spread beyond the prostate.

To determine the possible spread of the disease a variety of blood tests, bone scans, X-rays, CT scans, MRIs, ultrasounds and even lymph node biopsies may be done.

CONVENTIONAL TREATMENT OF PROSTATE CANCER

A detailed discussion of conventional prostate cancer is beyond the scope of this monograph. However, it is important to know that conventional treatment for prostate cancer is currently in transition. The basic protocol that has been used for years is currently being questioned for a number of reasons. These include: (1) Prostate cancer is a slow-growing disease, and it takes a long time to evaluate the effects of treatment. (2) Prostate cancer is often dormant for many years and many men who die of other causes have prostate cancer at autopsy without ever having known about it during their lifetimes. (3) Recent diagnostic techniques, such as the PSA, transrectal ultrasound of the prostate and the procedure using multiple biopsies of the prostate have resulted in both an increase in the diagnosis of prostate cancer and also earlier diagnosis. (4) The so-called curative procedure for prostate cancer, namely, radical prostatectomy, is a dangerous procedure, with many serious side effects that may significantly worsen the quality of life for its recipient, even though the cancer may be "cured." (5) For selected patients, recent modifications and improvements in surgical technique of the radical prostatectomy, namely, the nerve-sparing procedure developed by Dr. Walsh at Johns Hopkins, has significantly reduced the morbidity and mortality associated with radical prostate surgery, but it is unclear how many urologists are well trained in this method. (6)

Although newer, potentially curative and much less invasive and dangerous procedures, such as cryosurgery, are currently being used, they have not been available long enough to evaluate their effectiveness because of the long course of prostate cancer. (7) Between 25 and 50 percent of patients who are clinically diagnosed as having stages A2, B or C turn out to actually have stage D prostate cancer.

For all of these reasons, sometimes treatment is no more effective than watchful waiting. Willet F. Whitmore Jr., M.D., of Memorial Sloan-Kettering Cancer Center in New York, has asked: "Is cure possible in those for whom it is necessary and is cure necessary in those for whom it is possible?"[5]

Treatments

The current treatment recommended by most urologists for stages A and B prostate cancer is either radical prostatectomy or external beam radiation. Both treatments have significant side effects, and neither has been shown to be definitely effective in prospective randomized trials because of some of the reasons previously discussed. If they have any role to play, however, it is for stage A or B. These treatments are generally considered inappropriate for stages C and D. However, a recent survey found that more than half of stage C and stage D prostate cancer patients inappropriately received one of these treatments.

According to many prostate cancer experts, the most appropriate treatment for stage C or stage D prostate cancer is complete hormonal blockade. In this treatment, drugs are used to stop testosterone production and inhibit its effects. By totally ablating testosterone effects, the vast majority of advanced prostate cancer patients will have a remission of the disease for varying periods of time, some for several years. The drugs most frequently used are: (1) leuprolide (Lupron) which inhibits pituitary secretions that lead to testosterone production by the testes and (2) flutamide (Eulexin) which blocks testosterone from combining with its receptor protein, thus preventing any testosterone effect.

Although this treatment often results in regression of stage C and stage D prostate cancer for significant periods of time, the therapeutic effects usually wear off after awhile. The cancer cells appear to become hormone resistant, and the disease becomes very difficult to treat. The patient often dies a painful death with bony metastases within months to occasionally years of the time that the cancer becomes resistant to hormonal treatment.

A major controversy involving conventional treatment is a new protocol advocated by a prostate cancer patient advocacy group that disagrees with the majority of urologists. This group, Patient Advocates of Advanced Cancer Treatments (PAACT), with the backing of several physicians including oncologists, recommends at least a short course (six months to a year) of complete hormonal blockade for most early-stage prostate cancer patients followed, if necessary, by cryosurgery, a method of freezing any remaining cancerous tissue in the prostate. According to this group, this protocol involves many fewer side effects and risk to the patient.

Alternatively, they suggest that a course of complete hormonal blockade in the early stages of prostate cancer may downstage the disease, so that treatment with a radical prostatectomy will show better results than if the surgery were done immediately at the time of diagnosis. It is too early to tell whether this approach will prove to be better than the current approach of most urologists.

Complementary Prevention and Treatment

A complementary approach to preventing and treating prostate cancer can be very effective, just as it is for benign disorders of the prostate. In my opinion, all prostate cancer patients should incorporate complementary treatment approaches whether or not they also do conventional treatment. The complementary approach emphasizes removing toxic exposures and toxic substances from the body, nourishing the organ systems, including the immune system and generally strengthening the body so that one's own internal defenses can be mobilized to neutralize or rid the body of the prostate cancer. Among the methods used for this purpose are the dietary recommendations and "avoid list" previously discussed on pages 22–24, the nutritional supplements previously mentioned on pages 25–32, as well as others which are more specific for cancer.

In my own practice, we recommend a variety of herbs, such as the Essiac mixture, a mixture known as Vitae Elixxir and others. We also use high doses of certain nutrients, such as vitamin C and other antioxidants, in both oral and intravenous forms. Other substances useful for helping the body fight cancer include certain soybean extracts, shark cartilage and bovine cartilage. A useful nontoxic chemotherapy we sometimes recommend is hydrazine sulfate, and when the patient is able to obtain amygdalin (also known as Laetrile) we find this also to be useful, both orally and intravenously. Of course, other therapeutic recommendations previously discussed for treating BPH such diet, exercise and stress management should be part of a complemetary treatment program for prostate cancer.

Many of our prostate cancer patients appear to be preventing the worsening of their clinical prostate cancers by just using a combination of these complementary cancer treatments. For others, these methods are combined with one or more of the conventional treatments. Some patients with elevated PSAs and a transrectal ultrasound of the prostate suggestive of prostate cancer refuse to allow a biopsy and instead go on an intensive anticancer complementary program with careful monitoring of the PSAs and ultrasounds. Considering the fact that many prostate cancers never do become aggressive and that one treatment option even by conventional physicians is watchful waiting, this approach seems reasonable. Generally, men undergoing such a program feel an increased sense of well-being, often finding improvement in other medical problems. Negative side effects are usually none or very minor. The downside of such a program is the cost, time and effort required to implement such a program and the possibility of the disease worsening if the program doesn't work. This last possibility is best dealt with by careful monitoring and a flexible approach to changing the treatment if goals are not being accomplished.

A prostate cancer prevention program would incorporate most of the lifestyle recommendations, dietary suggestions, avoid list, exercise program and stress management programs previously described.

In addition, there is some evidence that hormonal balancing, including supplementing with testosterone when necessary, would help to prevent prostate cancer. In Dr. Debled's series of 2,000 men treated with testosterone over the past 15 to 20 years, one would have expected the development of clinical prostate cancer in at least 50 of them. He reports that none of his patients ever developed prostate cancer. This report tends to contradict conventional urological wisdom and needs to be confirmed. In the meantime, the fearful reluctance of most conventional urologists to supplement with testosterone appears to be unfounded.

In summary, a man trying to prevent prostate cancer or to treat it once it has been diagnosed would be wise to look into the complementary approach of non-toxic therapies.

REFERENCES

1. Coffey, D. S. The molecular biology, endocrinology, and physiology of the prostate and seminal vesicles. In: *Campbell's Urology*, 6th edition, Ed. by Walsh, P. C., Retik, A. B., et al., p. 225, W. B. Saunders: Harcourt Brace Jovanovich, Philadelphia, PA, 1992, p. 221.
2. Cassin, B. F., Pontes, J. E., Carcinoma and intraepithelia prostate in young male patients. *J Urol* 150 (2 Pt. 1): August 1993, 379–385.
3. Mann, C. C. The prostate-cancer dilemma. *The Atlantic Monthly*, November 1993, 102–118.
4. *Prostate Cancer Report* (4th edition), PAACT, Grand Rapids, MI, 1992, p. 12.
5. Salmans, Sandra. *Prostate: Questions you have ... Answers you need.* People's Medical Society, Allentown, PA, 1993, p. 128.